What's Up, Doc?

How to Get Your Doctor
to Really Listen to You

Glenn Miya, MD

Published by
Duswalt Press
280 N. Westlake Blvd
Suite 110
Westlake Village, CA 91362
www.duswaltpress.com

Manufactured in the United States of America, or in the
United Kingdom when distributed elsewhere.

Miya,Glenn
What's Up Doc? How to Get Your Doctor to Really Listen To You
ISBN:
Paperback: 9781938015359
eBook: 9781938015366

Cover design by: Joe Potter
Cover illustrator by: Dennis Auth
Interior design: Scribe Inc.
Permission credits: Dennis Auth

Disclaimer: The purpose of this book is to educate and entertain. The author
or publisher does not guarantee that anyone following the techniques,
suggestions, tips, ideas, or strategies will improve their health or their
relationship with their health care provider. This book is not meant to replace
the advice and recommendations of a person's own health care provider.

Names and characteristics of people in this book have been changed to
protect identities. Some characterizations are a composite of multiple cases
for the sake of protecting people's identities and for the sake of example.
Any resemblance to any real-life individual is purely coincidental.

Any mention of brand name medications and websites does not
imply endorsement or recommendation. The author and publisher
shall have neither liability nor responsibility to anyone with respect
to any loss or damage caused, or alleged to be caused, directly
or indirectly by the information contained in this book.

Author's URL: DrGlennMiya.com

Dedication

To my patients,

who have made me a better listener

Acknowledgments

The author would like to thank the following people for their time and support during the course of this project:

Steven Llanusa
Craig Duswalt
Andrew Pais
Karen Strauss
Ardis Weiss
Michael Stevenson
Kayla Stevenson
Jason Hughes
Rev. T. Michael Dawson
Dr. Paul Orr
Marcia Brandwynne
Sean Pilon

Contents

Contents

Introduction

WHY YOU NEED THIS BOOK

You need this book because you're busy and your doctor is busy.

Whether you spend an hour with your concierge physician or five minutes with a physician's assistant at a busy urgent care clinic, this book will help you make the most of your visit.

What is often overlooked is that doctors speak a foreign language. Sure, it may resemble your native tongue, but actually it is immersed in acronyms, Latin, medical jargon, idioms, and a cultural mind-set based on a template of problem solving called SOAP. (More on that later.) Don't worry. Unless you're already in the medical field, you don't have to learn doctor-speak.

Before I went to Milan for vacation, I didn't have time to take a course in Italian. I did learn a few phrases and customs, and I studied a map of the city from a pocket guide. I'm glad I did. I was met with polite smiles and helpful service, while my uninitiated travel buddy was met with misunderstanding.

That's what this book is: a guide to helping you get the most out of your doctor visits with a minimum of misunderstanding and wasted time.

But communication is a two-way street. You may be thinking, "Shouldn't doctors hold the burden of responsibility in making sure their communication with patients is crystal clear?" I can assure you that doctors themselves get training and continuing medical education credit for learning to improve their communication skills with patients. The courses emphasize active listening, empathy, compassion, and translating medical terms for easy understanding—in other words, acting like the normal, decent human beings they were before they suffered internship and their handwriting became hieroglyphics. My last training had lessons on when to smile. Doctors are trying to keep up their side of the bargain. This book will help you assist your doctor to do her job better, which is to diagnose, treat, and provide care. The better job a doctor does, the more you'll benefit.

Unfortunately, there is another reason for this book. The doctor-patient relationship is eroding. It is eroding from constraints on time, constraints on what insurance will allow, higher premiums, and lower reimbursements. Communication is the cornerstone of a viable doctor-patient therapeutic alliance on which accurate diagnosis, treatment, trust, and continuity of care depend. This book has tips to improve and streamline your communication with your physician.

DISCLAIMER

The purpose of this book is to educate and entertain. The author or publisher does not guarantee that anyone following the techniques, suggestions, tips, ideas, or strategies will improve their health or their relationship with their health care provider. This book is not meant to replace the advice and recommendations of a person's own health care provider. Names and characteristics of people in this book have been changed to protect identities. Some characterizations are a composite of multiple cases for the sake of protecting people's identities and for the sake of example. Any resemblance to any real-life individual is purely coincidental. Any mention of brand name medications and websites does not imply endorsement or recommendation. The author and publisher shall have neither liability nor responsibility to anyone with respect to any loss or damage caused, or alleged to be caused, directly or indirectly by the information contained in this book.

Before Your Visit

Finding a Doctor

If I were new in town and looking for a new primary physician, I would start with word-of-mouth recommendations. I'd ask my neighbors and colleagues whom they see. I'd ask how long they have been with their doctor. Most importantly, I would ask why they've chosen to stay with him or her. "What is it about this particular doctor that makes you trust him or her? How well do the two of you communicate?"

I would ask about the personalities of the physician, nurses, and office staff. I would also ask how the doctor handles after-hours calls.

I'm not against checking out a clinic's website or testimonials on the Internet. Keep in mind that there are great doctors who don't have or don't need websites to maintain their business. Testimonials can also be skewed, coming from the most satisfied or most dissatisfied of patients.

Interviewing for a Potential Doctor

While some consumer magazines recommend interviewing a doctor before signing up with one, there are two caveats to be aware of.

First, many doctors are so busy they don't have time to interview with potential patients for free. Be prepared to offer a cash price for their time.

Second, you may not get an accurate sense of the doctor's capabilities through an interview. The reason for this is that doctors are intrinsically detectives and problem solvers. An interview doesn't allow you to observe them in action—solving a problem, making a diagnosis, explaining a diagnosis, and creating a treatment plan. You could be interviewing a great diagnostician who just doesn't interview well with strangers when there's no problem to be solved. If you were a basketball coach, would you judge a player based on what he says he can do or your observation on how he actually performs on the court?

If you want to set up an initial get-to-know-each-other visit, be prepared. Have your past medical history and list of medications ready. Discuss how your conditions have been treated before and what your expectations are. One visitor I had brought in his old records that dealt with his hypothyroidism. He presumed I was trained in prescribing bioidentical hormones. I wasn't, but I referred the gentleman to a colleague who was.

Organize Your Medical Records

YOU HAVE ONE PATIENT: YOU

Depend on yourself, not your doctor or your chart, to record your medical history. Your doctor is busy. In some health maintenance organizations, a physician may be assigned more than 2,000 patients. He may see between 16 and 32 (or more) patients a day. Additionally, he has the duty to address phone calls, pharmacy refill requests, prior authorization requests, letters, disability forms, insurance forms, and chart audits—not to mention driving to the hospital to visit in-patients. Don't get me wrong. I'm sure he has a good memory of your past medical history and your chronic conditions like asthma and high blood pressure. But remember: Your doctor may have two thousand patients to look after. You have only one. (You may have more than one if you're a parent.)

Keep a Notebook

At the very least, you should keep a notebook. Fill it with dates when you visited the doctor and the reasons for the visits. Write down the medications you are taking now and the ones you took in the past. Keep a timeline of your past surgeries, injuries, hospitalizations, and allergic reactions to medications. Record your vaccinations and any important procedures you may have had done, such as colonoscopies or heart angiograms (a special x-ray that highlights your arteries with dye). Include your advance directive, stating who should make medical decisions on your behalf if you are unable to. Your notebook is also a good place to write down your family tree with the diseases and causes of death of your relatives. Were there any first-degree relatives with colon, breast, or ovarian cancer? Such information may determine if you need additional tests. Ask to get paper copies of your latest blood results, EKGs, x-rays, and consultation reports. These are especially important if you see multiple doctors. Bring your notebook to every doctor visit, including those with specialists.

Your Specialists Are Special

If you see specialists, keep a list of their names and phone numbers along with your primary doctor's contact information. I have patients who have two kidney specialists—one who is local and another who works at a major university center fifty miles away. An emergency room doctor needs to know which one to contact depending on the issue. Without a list of your doctors, you could be "lost to follow-up." One of my own patients was under the care of another doctor across town for heart failure for six months because the hospital discharged her to that doctor. She couldn't remember my name after receiving morphine.

Electronic Medical Records

If you have computer access, I recommend keeping electronic records. (One patient accidentally left his notebook of many years on the roof of his car. He later saw the contents of the notebook in his rearview mirror, strewn across four lanes of the freeway he was on.) There are many apps and websites, such as HealthVault.com, that will keep your information organized and secure. If you end up in an urgent care clinic and the doctor wants to compare your current EKG with one from two years ago, you can bring it up on your phone or a nearby computer. That old EKG alone may determine if you are to be hospitalized or discharged home.

Your doctor may use an electronic medical record program, such as Practice Fusion, that allows patients access to parts of their virtual chart. Some large health networks such as Kaiser Permanente allow patients access to their own health summaries and lab results. In any case, have access to an organized record of your past medical history. Your doctor will surely inquire into it. It will streamline the flow of information and reduce medical inaccuracies.

Put It in Your Wallet

Whether you put your records on paper or online, summarize your past medical history, allergic reactions, and medications to fit on a 3" × 5" card and keep it in your wallet along with your insurance card. You'll be glad you did (and the doctor will too) if you ever end up on a gurney in the emergency room.

Keep a List of Your Medications

Put your medicine bottles in a bag and bring them to your first visit. Your doctor will record them and check for redundancies and potential drug interactions. Bring any over-the-counter medications, vitamins, or herbs as well. Don't forget meds that are not pills—in other words, inhalers, creams, patches, eye drops, injections, and so on. They are *all* important to mention. Your doctor may take an inventory of your meds to check for possible drug-to-drug interactions, duplications, errors, and expiration dates. Ask your physician if she would prefer that you bring the bottles again or a list at subsequent visits.

I remember many times on-call when I would admit an unfamiliar patient from the emergency room. Having arrived by ambulance, the patient would have no record of his medications. A call home to the patient's wife at 3 a.m. on Saturday would lead to fumbling through the medicine cabinet followed by a groggy reciting of the spelling of each word on expired bottles' labels. All I needed was to know was one drug's name and dosage. I would finally get my answer when I spoke to the patient's primary doctor's nurse on Monday morning. Such inefficiency could be avoided.

Over-the-Counter Medications

In addition to prescriptions, all medications should be divulged to your doctor. This includes acetaminophen, aspirin, nonsteroidal anti-inflammatory medications, weight-loss meds, antihistamines, and hydrocortisone cream. Also included are herbal medications, vitamins, supplements, and Chinese medicines. I have patients who are taking medications bought in Mexico, and I ask them to bring them to the visit so I can inspect them.

Any medication that is strong enough to help you is strong enough to produce side effects or complications. Just because a medication can be store-bought does not mean it is safer than a prescription medication. Furthermore, herbal medicines are not FDA approved, so there is no formal routine for testing the efficacy, adverse effects, and drug-to-drug interactions of these meds.

For example, St. John's wort, which has been used to treat depression, can have a blood-thinning effect. One of my patients on St. John's wort had periods so heavy that she had to go to the emergency room to stop them.

A middle-aged man underwent several prostate exams, urinalyses, and blood tests before it was discovered that a "men's vitamin" was responsible for a strange, clear penile discharge.

Ma Huang or Ephedra, a stimulant, was banned by the FDA in 2004 after a number of deaths were linked to the drug.

I've seen two-year-olds become hyperactive after taking over-the-counter cough syrups meant for five-year-olds.

My point? When you bring in your medications, bring the bottles of *all* your medications.

Know What Your Insurance Covers

You can't ask for services until you know what services are covered.

The doctor-patient relationship is really a threesome. There's the patient, the doctor, and the insurance. Know what's covered and what's not. Each insurance is different. If your physician works for the Veteran's Administration (VA) or an all-in-one Health Maintenance Organization (HMO), then she is contracted with essentially one insurance type. Personally, I am contracted with multiple insurance companies. Each one has their own set of rules and regulations. There is no standardization. Some cover physical exams; others don't. Some cover vaccinations; others don't. Each has its own unique pharmacy formulary. Some require prior authorization for certain brand medications through an independent pharmaceutical mail-order company. Others require prior authorizations for MRIs through an independent radiological review company. Dealing with ten different insurance companies is like dealing with ten different types of currency!

Another reason to know exactly what your insurance covers has to do with the way billing occurs. Payments—and nonpayments—from billing the insurance are delayed. Let's say you would like to receive the Gardasil vaccine to prevent infections from the human papilloma virus (HPV). You aren't sure whether your insurance covers it and neither is the clinic staff, and they don't have time to call your insurance company to find out. You decide to get the vaccine anyway, and your doctor bills your insurance company. Two months later, the claim is denied because Gardasil is not a covered benefit, and you end up with the bill. It would have been wiser to know the cost of the vaccine and your covered benefits beforehand. Getting services without knowing if they are covered is like using your credit card to buy expensive clothes without a price tag. You won't find out the cost until you get the statement.

How to Talk to Your Doctor during Your Visit

Be Nice to the Staff

Your visit to the doctor starts when you enter the clinic. Be nice to the receptionists at the front desk. Be nice to the medical assistants and nurses checking you into the room. Be nice to the medical biller. They may all be your lifeline in an emergency.

The entire staff most likely has been schooled on the necessity of patient confidentiality, from insurance issues to private health matters. Don't hesitate to discuss issues with the staff. Some people wait until they are in the examination room to vent everything from their frustration being in the waiting room to their ingrown toenail. This wastes valuable time. Have a question or complaint? Start with the front-desk staff and they will direct your concerns to the right staff member.

Start with the Chief Complaint

Finally you're in the examination room with the doctor. Bring a list of your top two or three symptoms or concerns and start with the most pressing one first. That first concern you broach is called the chief complaint, and it guides me in my line of questioning. If you have pain, be prepared to succinctly answer the following questions:

How long have you had it?
How would you describe it?
Where is it exactly?
Is it continuous, or does it ever go away?
What makes it better?
What makes it worse?
What are you usually doing when it is at its worst?
What have you tried at home already to alleviate it?
What other symptoms go along with it?
How would you rate the pain on a scale of one to ten?

Be Descriptive

If you have a headache, for example, provide me with descriptive details. Doctors are listening for telltale classic descriptions of certain diagnoses. Telling me that it's your worst headache ever or that the pain is like "an ice pick in the left eye" or that the headache came on strong and quick like a loud clap in the head may help me discern a mild condition from one that is life threatening.

Tell Me the Sequence of Your Symptoms

Doctors understand the evolution of disease. For example, in adults, appendicitis may start off with mild upper, midabdominal pain that later moves to the right-lower quadrant of the belly and becomes more intense. That's a different description than saying, "Hey Doc, I've got sharp pain on my lower right side whenever I walk, over the last month." Or, do you have sinus pain, a runny nose, and a fever? It matters to me if the fever came before or after the sinus pain. Tell me your symptoms in the *order* they happened.

No "Hand-on-the-Doorknob" Questions

I cannot impress enough how critical it is to start with the most important, most pressing, most distressing symptom first. All doctors dislike the "hand-on-the-doorknob" question. That's the question that a patient asks just at the close of the visit, when the doctor places his hand on the doorknob before escorting the patient out of the room. It often turns out to be the most important reason for the visit in the first place. Some of the doorknob questions I have received are the following:

> "I have been having squeezing chest pain every time I walk. Can you just check my heart?"
> "By the way, I have been hearing voices. Is that OK?"
> "I found a new lump on my rump. Can you take a peek?"
> "I have been having night sweats for the last month."

Last-minute chief complaints are exasperating. They can also be dangerous. Leaving a chief complaint for the last minute may change the entire crux or even the diagnosis of your visit. Each visit is choreographed with a conversation first, a physical examination next, a discussion of the diagnosis at hand, and then a review of the treatment plan. For example, symptoms of back pain may elicit a set of possible muscular ailments in the doctor's mind. But back pain plus night sweats could mean something much more serious in the categories of infection or cancer. Don't waste time by leaving your chief complaint hanging on the doorknob.

Be Candid and Be Brief

I ask my patients to read all three of their concerns first because they may all be interrelated. For example, a fifty-year-old woman may have three new symptoms of heart palpitations, insomnia, and joint pain. Further questioning on my part will determine if these are three independent conditions or three symptoms related to perimenopause. Doctors are trained to look for an "economy of diagnosis"—in other words, a constellation of attributes that will lead to a unifying diagnosis.

If you are symptom-free and are at the visit for your annual physical exam, I would like to hear about any pertinent changes since our last visit:

Did you visit other doctors?
Has there been a change in your list of medications?
Have you been sick or injured?

I'm also interested in any major life changes that may be affecting your health including the death of loved one, a change in marital status, a change of residence, or even a change of insurance. If you didn't take your medications as prescribed, let me know the reason. I assure my patients that they are not in the principal's office, but conversing with a doctor is part confessional, part courtroom testimony. Be candid and brief.

Here's a nice sheet to organize your visit that was created by Rev. M. Thomas Dawson:

CLINIC VISIT INFORMATION WORKSHEET

Name _____ Date _____

The first problem I've come to see you about today is:

_____

_____

_____

_____

_____

My symptoms are:

_____

_____

_____

_____

_____

The second problem I've come to see you about today is:

_____

_____

_____

_____

_____

My symptoms are:

_____

_____

_____

_____

_____

(continued)

Medications:

Name	Dose	Times per day	Is a refill needed?

Allergies:

Drug	Reaction

Designed by T. Michael Dawson

Be Explicit

No matter how embarrassing the subject may be, I reassure my patients that they can tell me anything. I have heard it all. And if I haven't heard it before, I promise I won't laugh, criticize, judge, or be shocked. Getting the right medical care demands being blunt. But trust me, I can handle it. I'm a doctor. Doctors have been through internship and residency, a boot camp of blood, sweat, tears, and a lot of other secretions from every orifice of the body. We're not squeamish. We have seen more gore than there is in a Wes Craven trilogy. We have delivered babies and delivered bad news. We have counseled kids on chemotherapy. We have talked to psychotics. We have seen the moment of death occur before our eyes.

So whatever it is, just tell the doctor. Many of my male patients who come in for erectile dysfunction lie to my nurse when she does her intake interview. She leaves the room and then I come in. At this point they say, "Doc, I told the nurse I'm here because of a sore throat, but I'm really here because I want to talk about Viagra." Giving misleading information is confusing and it wastes time. Whatever notes the nurse has already written in the chart become part of a legal document, and the doctor must edit it and redirect his note taking. Also, auditors from insurance companies routinely review doctors' chart notes for consistency and completeness. Misleading information won't help your doctor.

No Subject Is Taboo

I've known persons to withhold pertinent information about sex, masturbation, homosexuality, prostitution, drug abuse, spousal abuse, seeing delusions, hearing voices, rape, incest, nightmares, suicidal thoughts, depression, cutting, bulimia, genital warts, criminal history, and many other topics. In each case, the delay in divulging critical information led to a delay in proper diagnosis and treatment. Life coach Rick Clemons has said that any information that you withhold could put your doctor at a disadvantage in being able to assist you.

In short, whatever's bugging you, just say it! And if you can't say it, write it down.

Don't Pre-diagnose Yourself

Any medical problem that's troubling you enough to scour the Internet is worth having a professional carefully diagnose.

Why?

There's no computer yet invented that will outsmart a human doctor like that computer on *Jeopardy*.

Medical websites are meant to convey information on conditions—not to diagnose. The verbal descriptions and visual depictions are classic textbook examples. They usually characterize a disease in its most robust, most delineated, unequivocal state. In real life, illnesses are usually not so clear and are witnessed in their early, more nebulous state. A doctor is trained to look for atypical presentations of common diseases as well as typical presentations of uncommon diseases.

One pediatrician said it best when it comes to medical websites: "There is too much information out there." There is also misinformation. I don't mind my patients doing research on their symptoms before their visit—in fact, I appreciate it. What I don't appreciate is a patient blurting out a diagnosis at the beginning of a visit.

Physicians themselves are sometimes the worst patients. While they speak the same language as the practitioner, they often greet the doctor saying, "I'm sure I have bronchitis. I need some antibiotics." They think they're helping out their own doctor by cutting to the chase. In essence, they are doing themselves a disservice. Why? Because by virtue of being sick, a person has blind spots. A patient may feel a "little tired" while suffering a heart attack. I've witnessed that. A child may have a high fever and look perfectly content. Sometimes appendicitis can mimic a stomach flu. I myself went to the ER when I thought I was a having a bad migraine. It turned out to be viral meningitis. I learned my lesson. A sick person diagnosing himself or herself is akin to performing an appendectomy on oneself. The condition itself may obscure your perspective.

Give your doctor the courtesy of listening to your history of symptoms, performing a hands-on examination, reviewing test results, and then making a diagnosis. That's his job as he methodically follows the SOAP approach.

What's SOAP?

SOAP stands for Subjective, Objective, Assessment, Plan. It's the four-part format by which doctors are trained to assess every clinical problem. *Subjective* refers to the patient's description of her ailment. It is the patient's personal interpretations, such as "My stomach pain is sometimes sharp, like a knife." *Objective* refers to the findings on the physical exam—indifferent to the doctor's or patient's opinion. The doctor may write in his note, "The abdomen was soft and nontender to palpation (pressing down)." Lab results also fall under the rubric of the objective. *Assessment* is the diagnosis deduced from the subjective and the objective information. Finally, the *plan* is the course of action: a prescription, a change in medicine, a referral to a specialist, or perhaps running additional tests to confirm the assessment.

SOAP is the way we physicians analyze what we see, hear, and touch in the clinic room. It is the format by which we write our notes in the clinic and in the hospital. They are often called SOAP notes. It is the order of information presented to us on board exams that test our detective abilities. It is the way physicians from different specialties communicate with each other when they are consulting on the same patient. It is the way medical students nervously communicate to their redoubtable attending physician when they have two minutes to present a case in the ER. SOAP is a format, a language, and a mindset. If you as the patient understand that doctors are filtering everything through SOAP, you can efficiently get your doctor to listen to you.

Cut the Small Talk

Most of my patients are well trained by my nurse. By the time I enter the examining room, they are sitting on the exam table, ready to blurt out their chief complaint, and partially clothed, with a drape sheet over the part of the body that needs to be checked. There's a handshake and a smile before we get down to business. It's not that we're being impersonal. Quite the opposite. We're both getting right to the heart of their most personal matter: their health.

Small talk is breaking the ice, shooting the breeze, and chewing the fat. It's fine for strangers at cocktail party, but it just wastes time in the doctor's office. While I appreciate your asking how my three children are, I know that you really want to find out why you are having indigestion and how you can prevent it.

Ask the Tough Questions

As your visit with the doctor comes to a close, she may be writing a prescription or recommending a treatment plan. If you don't agree with the plan, now is the time to speak up!

- If a medicine is being prescribed, ask what the side effects may be. Ask what would happen if you choose not to take the medication. Ask if there is a cheaper alternative.
- If surgery or an invasive procedure is recommended, ask what all your options are. Ask if you can delay making your decision. Ask if you can get a second opinion or where you can research more information.
- If you are referred to a consultant, ask why the consultant is needed. Ask if the consultant is one the doctor would entrust his family with.
- If no specific treatment is prescribed, ask why. What symptoms should you be watching for? Who should you call if your condition worsens?
- If you have any questions about your condition, ask if you can get information to read.
- If tests are being performed, ask what the doctor is looking for specifically. Ask how the results may change the plan of action. Ask if the tests are covered by the insurance.

Second Opinion versus Another Opinion

A word about second opinions. Most doctors are not indignant if a patient requests a second opinion. If a life-or-death disease like cancer is diagnosed, it is not unusual for an oncologist to offer a second opinion, especially when multiple treatment options are being considered. In other instances, however, getting a second opinion may be a little complicated.

I counsel my patients that if they seek a second opinion that they are clear on the terminology that they use. For example, if Doctor A recommends surgery and the patient seeks a second opinion from Doctor B, it is implied that Doctor B will give his advice, and then the patient will return to Doctor A for continuation of care. Some doctors don't like giving second opinions for a variety of reasons. Some may feel indignant that they were not asked first. Some may feel uncomfortable disagreeing with their colleague. If the patient, however, states that he is seeking Doctor B for "another opinion," then after Doctor B gives his advice, the patient may choose to go with Doctor A or Doctor B for continuation of care.

Be Blunt

If you feel there is a breakdown in communication, speak up. You have a professional relationship with your doctor. This is not a time to worry about hurting feelings (Avitzur).

> "Doctor, I am not sure I am getting my message across."
> "I don't understand."
> "Say it in plain English."
> "I need you to repeat that and write it down."

Once, after returning twenty minutes late from the hospital on my lunch break, I bolted into an exam room. I said I was sorry for the delay as I was flipping through a chart while ruminating about my pediatric patient in the intensive care unit. My longtime octogenarian patient told me to sit down, slow down, and calm down. I'm glad he did. I could listen to him clearly now.

Keep Notes

Document your visit. Often there is a lot of information to absorb. Have the diagnosis and treatment plan written down by you or the doctor. Ask questions to clarify. Alternatively, you may want a friend or relative in the room as your advocate and note-taker. Some patients audio record their visits with the doctor's permission. Consider asking for brochures, books, or websites where you can find additional information.

Kids Comfort

School-age kids normally get embarrassed about undressing at the doctor's office. Some refuse to wear a gown. Others are afraid to be touched. I know twin seven-year-olds who scream every time they are in my office—and that's before I even enter the room! While most parents do their best to explain calmly what's expected of them prior to the visit, inevitably some kids can get the fight, flight, or freeze response when it's time to actually be examined.

I sometimes distract children with toys, balloons, and floor play. If the child is small enough, I let the parent hold him in her arms or on her lap while I'm looking in his ears or placing my stethoscope on his chest. A fellow pediatrician of mine had the brilliant idea of having her shy youngsters wear bathing suits at their well visits. The kids suddenly became as excited about going to the doctor's office as they were about going to the beach.

When kids are comfortable at the doctor's office, they are more apt to interact with the doctor and build rapport.

Between Visits

Update Your Records

Between visits, I recommend reviewing your notes and updating your medical notebook, whether it's on paper or on a computer. Notify your doctor if you experience severe side effects or a failure of medications. If there is a problem at night, know the number to call for after-hours advice. Know which urgent care clinic or emergency room to visit. In any case, unless your doctor gives you permission, I don't recommend calling him at home or showing up on his doorstep at 11 p.m.

No Curbside Consults

Among physicians, there's a difference between a formal consult and a curbside consult. When a primary care doctor calls a specialist to formally visit a patient in the hospital, it is called a formal consult. For example, an internal-medicine doctor has a patient in the hospital with pneumonia that is not improving. She may request a consult from an infectious disease (ID) specialist. The ID consultant reviews the progress notes, visits the patient, and then writes or dictates a formal consultation report replete with recommendations on how to optimize the plan of treatment. The report becomes part of the patient's hospital record. The consultant bills the insurance for her work and gets paid for her expertise.

A curbside consult is informal and off the record. The same internist might flag down the ID specialist as she's walking down the hospital corridor, pull her aside, and ask her a quick question—"Doc, can I get a curbside consult?"—alerting the specialist that she needn't visit the patient and compose a formal report. "Should I order azithromycin or ampicillin-sulbactam for my patient's pneumonia?" The specialist gives her answer and saunters off to finish her rounds.

Well-meaning patients sometimes ask their doctor for "curbside consults." I don't recommend that. Here are some examples.

> A father brings in Jimmy, his five-year-old son, for an evaluation for a sore throat and an earache. After I finish the exam and write a prescription, the father asks, "Doctor, can you *just* look in my throat too? I think I'm coming down with the same thing. I don't have insurance."
> During a busy day in the clinic, I am racing from room to room. I'm walking and reading a chart at the same time. Judy, a patient of mine without an appointment, stops me as I'm heading into a room. "I *just* have a quick question." She tells me that her headaches are getting worse and asks what she should do.

My neighbor, Eric, is in my doorway in the dim light at 11 p.m. clutching his right elbow: "Can you *just* look at this? I might have broken a bone."

A stranger at my own dinner party cornered me in a hallway and proceeded to complain that he disagreed with own doctor's diagnosis of genital herpes from earlier that day: "Doc can you *just* take a quick look now?" Taken aback, I calmly reply, "I think it's best you talk to your doctor directly." (My snide colleague sarcastically suggested I should have answered, "Sure. Do you want me to check you out before or after I prepare tonight's sushi?")

In each of the previous examples, the patient said that red-flag word: "just." When I hear "just," I stop and realize that a patient's request is not "just" simple. It is risky for a patient to ask for a curbside consult, even if the doctor complies.

- A doctor could be held liable for informal advice.
- You're asking for free advice. You'll get what you pay for. You're also demeaning the value of your doctor's service.
- You're asking for advice on the fly. Your doctor may have something else on his mind and may not give your issue proper consideration.

In the first three cases, I could have easily stopped to handle the question at hand. However, I must admit that the context and my frame of mind would not have been optimal. What if Jimmy's father's throat condition needed an urgent ear, nose, and throat consultation? Am I now responsible for this patient? What if I were too busy to realize that Judy's headache was a red flag for a tumor? What if Eric's arm had a hairline fracture only visible on x-ray? I believe that if you are truly seeking a professional solution to a medical problem, then you deserve to have a physician's full attention in a clinical setting—with good lighting and proper instruments. Anything less is cutting corners.

In the last case, the dinner-party guy was crossed off my guest list for eternity.

Keep Your Doctor as Your Doctor, Not as Your Friend

Some of my closest friends have asked me to be their physician. My standard response has been, "I can be your doctor or I can be your friend. I cannot be both." Drawing the line between a professional and social relationship is an essential duty for both doctor *and* patient. Without the separation, conflict of interest can dilute and complicate the therapeutic alliance of the patient and doctor. Merriam-Webster's dictionary defines conflict of interest as "a conflict between the private interests and the official responsibilities of a person in a position of trust."

The difficulty lies in defining what a "friend" is. American culture does not have a hierarchy of distinction for friendship. If there were one, it might look something like this:

Confidante
Best friend forever
Best friend for now
Very good friend with whom I go to the gym and who knows part of my personal life
Very good friend whose company I enjoy for dinner (but only dinner)
Good friend who is fun and whom I call once in a while
Good friend whom I text
Friend with whom I go to social events
Friend I see at social events
Acquaintance I see at social events who sends holiday greeting cards every year
Acquaintance who sometimes sends a holiday greeting card
Acquaintance whom I barely remember but who is not weird and befriended me on Facebook

Where does one draw the line?

I know one doctor in a small town who won't speak or make eye contact with his patients when he sees them walking down the same aisle in the grocery store. He does this to keep private their professional relationship. Some patients don't want to be seen with any doctor outside of a medical context. He also does this to prevent the start of any social relationship.

I don't recommend making a friend your doctor or a doctor your friend. Friends play by a different set of rules. Friends don't like to criticize each other. Friends tend to agree. Friends have expectations of and obligations to each other. Friends are biased. A doctor should have objectivity in making judgments. A doctor who is a friend is liable to err in providing too much or too little treatment.

The line between friendship and doctor should be clear so a conflict of interest does not enter the relationship.

Don't Give, but If You Insist, Be Cheap

Doctors themselves have debated over the ethics of receiving gifts from patients. Some argue a doctor-patient relationship is a fiduciary relationship (Weijer). Thus, gifts are unnecessary and could invite conflicts of interest in the mind of the doctor or patient—or both. A doctor may feel obligated to provide preferential treatment to the patient who provides a gift. Or the patient may expect preferential treatment.

On the other hand, other doctors feel that receiving an inexpensive token of appreciation is being polite and will not affect their sense of judgment or perception of the patient (Anderek). Both sides agree that expensive gifts are not appropriate because of the appearance of quid pro quo.

If your doctor accepts gifts, experts recommend that both parties examine the reason behind giving and receiving the gift (Gaufberg). Is the doctor accepting the gift so as not to offend the giver? Is the patient giving a gift with the hope of receiving VIP treatment? It has been observed that patients who give gifts get *more* treatment but not necessarily *better* treatment.

If you feel the need to show your appreciation to your doctor, what then would constitute an inexpensive gift? A box of chocolates? Most of my colleagues agree that no material item is expected. What is most gratifying is a heartfelt letter of thanks (*Ask an MD*).

One of my patients sent me a handwritten letter thanking me for assisting her out of a panic attack one year ago. The letter was part of her "one-year anniversary" celebration, as she had made significant changes in her job, marriage, diet, and exercise plan after that one incident. I keep that letter framed, and it makes me feel gratified that I'm a physician.

Please Don't Ask for Favors

Asking your physician for gifts, services, or donations unrelated to your health care may also invite conflicts of interest. I'm referring to requests such as walk-a-thon donations, volunteering, or in-kind donations to your local elementary school play. Requests and favors may also subtly influence their perception of you.

Jake was a college student and an aspiring writer. He also experimented with street drugs. Because I'm in Toastmasters, he asked me if I would review his latest essay. At first I said yes; it was an innocuous request. Later that day, I called him and said no. It might affect the way we would interact with each other in the future. Suppose I gave him a harsh critique. Would he be forthcoming with his drug use later on? Suppose I gave him a glowing review. Would I begin to act like a mentor or become lenient with his drug abuse just because he was a good student? I explained to Jake that I wanted to have just one relationship with him—that of his physician. Our conversations since then have been unfettered.

Consultations with Specialists

While communicating concisely with your primary physician is important, it's even more crucial with specialists to whom you've been referred for a consultation. They don't have the luxury of a relationship with you built over time. They don't know your personality and nuances. Yet they are expected to help you with *one* condition in a short amount of time.

Why do primary care physicians make referrals in the first place? There are many reasons, such as the following:

- A baffling condition needs to be diagnosed.
- A suspected diagnosis needs to be confirmed.
- The diagnosis at hand is outside of the scope and expertise of the primary physician who is relying on the specialist for further guidance.
- A sophisticated procedure (e.g., colonoscopy, sleep study test, a biopsy, open heart surgery) or a specialized treatment (e.g., chemotherapy for cancer) is needed.

I often deal with patients who are befuddled after their experience with a specialist. This is not because the specialist did or said anything wrong, but usually because time ran out and the patient wasn't able to get their issues addressed fully. Being prepared before the visit will save time and disappointment.

Mary had a headache for one month, an earache for one week, and a long history of snoring. When the ENT (ear, nose, and throat) specialist point-blank asked, "Why are you here?" She replied passively, "I'm not really sure. My primary doctor sent me here." At this point, the specialist is frustrated that he will have to start from scratch to unravel a medical mystery. When did her symptoms start? What medications did she take? Which ones worked and which ones didn't? Were any tests done?

The ENT doctor examines her ears, nose, and throat and concludes that her headaches and earaches are related to allergies. He provides her with a corticosteroid nasal spray, an antihistamine, and instructions to follow up with her primary physician. As Mary is about to exit the exam room, she turns and asks, "And what are we going to do about my snoring? My doctor thinks my snoring has something to do with my headaches. I already knew that I have allergies." Dr. ENT shouts back, "Well if you knew that from the beginning, why didn't you say so up front? Checking for sleep apnea takes a longer time to diagnose correctly. It takes a different set of questions and a detailed questionnaire. You've wasted my time and now I'm behind schedule and I'm too frustrated to answer any more questions!" . . . *in his mind.* After fumbling for his composure, Dr. ENT asks Mary to schedule a follow-up visit and brusquely says, "We'll handle your snoring at your next visit." Then he's gone.

When Mary returns to me, she complains that Dr. ENT gave her "some meds," appeared rude, and didn't do anything for her headaches. She then requests another referral to a different specialist.

Sleep apnea is a condition in which the body essentially isn't getting enough oxygen at night. The patient snores loudly, stops breathing periodically, and feels unrefreshed during the day. This is sometimes accompanied by high blood pressure, headaches, and fatigue. In Mary's case, she also grinds her teeth at night (bruxism), causing jaw pain and earaches.

Such an encounter with a specialist could have turned out more productively if the reason for the consultation was boiled down to *one* simple question.

One simple question: Do I have sleep apnea?

That question should be written out on your paper referral to the consultant. If you don't see it, ask. Sometimes it might be written out in doctor language: "rule out sleep disorder," "needs sleep study for OSA (obstructive sleep apnea)," or just the main symptoms, "snoring and headaches."

What are some other typical questions specialists deal with? Depending on the specialty it could be one of the following:

- Is this a hernia or a groin strain?
- Do I need surgery for my gallstones?

- What's the cause of my recurrent chest pain?
- I've had seizures for five years, but they're becoming more frequent. What are my treatment options?
- I'm depressed, and three different medications have failed. What should I do now?
- Is this dark spot on my back cancer?
- Ten years ago I had a normal colonoscopy. Do I need another one?

What else would have helped?

A written timeline of when Mary's symptoms arose and how they were treated at the time

A current list of medications

A past history of any surgeries or conditions related to the ear, nose, and throat

The results of relevant blood tests, x-rays, CT scans, or prior consults (also called a "work-up")

With the goal in mind of answering one question, Dr. ENT would have reviewed the work-up, done his exam, and then recommended the next step in the work-up: an overnight sleep study. This is a test where Mary's behavior, sleep stages, blood pressure, blood oxygen, and other vital signs would be observed to rule in or rule out a diagnosis of a sleep disorder. She might even be considered a candidate for a tonsillectomy.

Every specialist I've encountered has appreciated a concise summary of the patient's current symptoms relative to their specialty. A cardiologist wants to hear a description of your chest pain, not how your knees hurt. An orthopedic surgeon wants to hear about how long you have had pain and swelling in your left knee, but not necessarily all of your other joints. Why? Because he only operates on one joint at a time! A rheumatologist, however, would be interested in knowing if you've had pain and swelling in any of your joints—knees, ankles, wrists, elbows, shoulders, and spine. Rheumatologists are bone and joint specialists too, but they don't perform joint operations. They examine the constellation of all your joints to see if there is an underling unifying diagnosis, such as rheumatoid arthritis or lupus.

Don't be miffed if a neurosurgeon is interested in hearing about your headaches but not your stinging chronic lower-back pain that shoots down to your right foot (sciatica). Both conditions are within her scope of practice, but time and sometimes rules from insurance constrain what can be covered in one visit. Here are some tips for visiting with specialists:

When seeing an ophthalmologist, it's important that you have a good timeline of events: when your symptoms started, why you think they started, what medications or treatments have already been tried, and whether or not you have seen an optometrist or any other specialists. Bring all your medications. Bring an update of any conditions that you may have, such as high blood pressure and diabetes, and any optometrist's reports.

Bring bottles of eye drops and any over-the-counter medications. Bring your most current pair of eyeglasses as well.

If you're seeing a neurologist or neurosurgeon, they will often want to have a scan such as a CT or MRI of the brain and/or spine before seeing you. Recent blood work would be helpful as well.

Electroencephalograms, which check seizure activity, and lumbar punctures are usually done at the request of the neurologist after the consultation if needed.

If you're seeing an ear, nose, and throat doctor (or otolaryngologist) or allergist, bring any past audiogram or tympanogram reports with you which reflect your ability to hear. If you had any allergy testing, bring copies of those. Bring any previous x-rays of the sinuses or scans of head and neck.

Have you seen another specialist for the same or similar issues such as a neurologist? Bring reports of that as well. These will all save time and make your appointment go much more efficiently.

For a cardiologist, past EKGs, past treadmill stress tests, emergency room reports, x-rays, and CAT scans of the chest are important. It goes without saying to bring your list of medications and a timeline of the events leading up to the visit.

A little secret here, there are some key elements that a cardiologist will ask with regards to the description of your chest pain.

Describe your chest pain. Was it dull? Sharp? Pressing? Where was it? In the middle of the chest? On the left side? Or on the right side? Did it radiate to the arm? To the left shoulder or left arm or to the neck or to the jaw?

With your finger, draw a circle around the area where you
had the chest pain. Was it in one small point, on the ribs,
or in a big general area over the left part of the chest?

What were you doing when the chest pain happened? What
are the things that make it worse, such as exercise or
eating? What are the things that make it better, such as
rest? What associated symptoms did you have with it?
Shortness of breath? Nausea? Vomiting? Cold, clammy
sweat? What time of the day did this happen? Are you
having any heartburn?

There are seven major risk factors for heart disease that
you will be asked about. They are high blood pressure,
diabetes, high cholesterol, having a parent with a
heart attack early in life, and cigarette smoking. (Being
male and advanced age are the last two risk factors.)

*It's especially important that you bring the results of your last
cholesterol reading.*

If you're going to be seeing a gastroenterologist, it's, again, important
to be very descriptive with your symptoms. Are you having any
abdominal pain? If so, during what part of the day? Does it happen
at night? Does it happen after a meal? If so, how long after a meal?

*How would you describe your abdominal pain? Is it sharp and
continuous? Is it burning? Is it dull? Does it restrict movement?*

*Bring a diet diary of what you've been eating and drinking. What
are your bowel habits? How often do you have a bowel movement?
Do you have any staining? Is there any blood in your stool? What
are your bowel movements like? Do they have a shape, size, and
consistency of a banana, or are they more like pellets?*

*What other symptoms are you having? Any nausea? Any diarrhea?
Fever? Weight loss? Does the abdominal pain radiate through the
back? Are you having any back pain? Are there certain foods that
trigger your abdominal discomfort, such as caffeine, spicy foods,
fast or greasy foods, or alcohol?*

If you're seeing a kidney specialist or nephrologist, bring the results of
kidney ultrasounds, kidney stone analyses, CAT scans, and chemistry
panels. Some would like to see 24-hour urine studies, which check for
kidney function and output of the calcium and protein in the urine.
A two-week diet diary would be helpful as well to see if you're eating

something that may be contributing to the formation of kidney stones. Include what your water intake is, what your caffeine intake is, and what your alcohol intake is.

For an orthopedic doctor or a rheumatologist, x-rays of the bones and joints in question are essential to bring, as well as any past medications used.

A rheumatologist would be interested in knowing if you've had a complete blood count, urinalysis, and possibly blood tests, including an ESR, CRP, ANA, rheumatoid fracture, HLA-B27, CPK, anti-DNase, or anti-Smith. Such sophisticated tests don't make or break a diagnosis but may aid in the diagnostic process. Have there been any rashes? If so, bringing photos would be helpful.

For a dermatologist, I recommend taking pictures of the rash. This could be done with a high-definition camera. Why photos? Photos are helpful in showing the evolution of the rash *prior* to your appointment with the dermatologist. For example,

Sometimes after using partially effective hydrocortisone cream, qualities of the rash itself may change and thus obfuscate the diagnosis. Scratching also alters the appearance of the rash thus making a diagnosis more difficult. Photos can help make a diagnosis before the rash became altered.

The dermatologist will also want to know if you've had any other major medical issues going on, such as diabetes, high blood pressure, liver disease, or allergies.

There are many other kinds of specialists that I have not listed here. If in doubt about what to bring to the visit, call and ask their office beforehand and the nurse or receptionist will let you know.

WHAT KIND OF SPECIALIST AM I BEING REFERRED TO?

It's imperative to know what kind of specialist you are being referred to. You'll better understand what types of treatment a given specialist can offer: surgery versus medication, for example.

Some parts of the body are handled by two types of specialists: one surgical and the other nonsurgical, or medical. For example, orthopedists are bone and joint surgeons while rheumatologists treat bones and joints with medications. Neurosurgeons perform brain and spinal surgery. Neurologists handle brain and spine conditions without surgery. Urologists are surgeons of the bladder and kidneys. Nephrologists treat the kidneys with medications or sometimes dialysis.

There are also some specialists who are trained in both the surgical and medical aspects: gynecologists and obstetricians (OB-GYN), dermatologists, and ophthalmologists, for example.

Finally, there are some specialties that don't have an exact surgical counterpart. Endocrinologists are hormone and metabolism experts, for example. There are also specialists in the immune system, infectious disease, and genetics. Specialties overlap too. As a woman, you can see a gynecologist or a urologist for recurrent bladder infections. And some consultants in pain management and PM&R (physical medicine and rehabilitation) get training in a variety of specialties—neurology, anesthesia, and orthopedics—to handle complex conditions such as chronic pain and rehabilitation from disability.

General surgeons handle everything from skin biopsies to dealing with almost any organ from the neck to the rectum. What they can't handle, they will refer to a surgeon who specializes in the heart, lung, colon, breast, or other organ.

If you're being referred to a hematologist (or blood specialist), please keep in mind that the doctor is known as a hematologist/oncologist (cancer specialist) or heme/onc for short. All doctors who are trained in blood disorders are also trained in cancer. That's because some blood diseases are blood cancers too (e.g., leukemia). I forgot to mention this distinction to Jim.

Jim had a rare type of anemia that I wanted a blood doctor to treat. When Jim checked in at the blood specialist's office, he was surprised to see patient brochures about cancer in the waiting area. There were also magazines about cancer. There were certificates on the wall displaying the doctor's competence in treating cancer. There were other patients who checked in at the receptionist's desk and said, "I'm here for my chemo."

The day after the consultation, Jim called me panicked. "Why did you send me to a cancer doctor? Do I really have cancer? What are you not telling me?" He was much relieved when I explained to him that blood specialists are cancer specialists, too, and that he did not have cancer.

Communicating
after the Visit

Pick Up the Phone

Ask your doctor how and when she would like to communicate in between visits. If you typically call in, leave a clear message or question with the receptionist. Ask how and when you will be notified about lab results. No news doesn't mean good news. Find out what your results are. Get clarification on results you don't understand.

Also, "normal" results don't always imply everything's OK. If an ultrasound of your abdomen comes back as normal but you are still having intestinal pain, then obviously something is still wrong. There are illnesses that might not show up on an ultrasound. Ask your doctor what should be done next.

To E-Mail or Not to E-Mail

Some malpractice insurance companies have warned doctors not to use electronic mail due to numerous liability issues. There are a number of reasons: A patient's e-mail may be overlooked or accidentally deleted. Or, if the doctor only checks his e-mail sporadically, there may be a critical delay in response to an emergency. Or, an e-mail may provoke the doctor to write a prescription without a hands-on, good-faith physical examination, putting the physician at risk for mistakes in judgment, diagnosis, and treatment. That doesn't serve you.

Sometimes patients make appointments to discuss things that don't require an exam. Wouldn't e-mail be more efficient you may ask? Maybe not. For example, one patient of mine needed help filling out his questionnaire for a confusing life insurance application. He wanted clarification on the medical terms in the application. While I could have answered online, I appreciated the fact that he valued my time and knowledge to ask me for a formal appointment. I answered his questions. I explained that "heart failure" doesn't mean cardiac arrest and so on. I translated some medical jargon. We reviewed his medical history so he was able to report it accurately. He got done in fifteen minutes what would have taken him hours with only the aid of the Internet and a medical dictionary.

On the other hand, e-mail has many advantages, and some large health care systems encourage its use to communicate with their doctors for prescription refills, appointment requests, and for reviewing lab results—no more waiting on hold with the receptionist. Some doctors rely on e-mail to keep them apprised of a patient's blood pressure readings or blood sugar readings—assuming that everything else is fine. An update may be helpful too. Once a patient sent me a missive while she was on vacation in Paris. She was treated by a French physician for a minor skin infection. There wasn't anything for me to do. I appreciated the note, as I was ready with appropriate follow-up care when she returned to see me.

To e-mail or not to e-mail? Talk it over with your physician and set clear and definite guidelines in writing. Your doctor may ask you to agree with such guidelines with your signature.

Social Media

I like Facebook. I just don't recommend it as a channel of communication with your doctor. The key word here is "social." If you befriend your doctor, you might be exposed to parts of his life about which you don't care to know. Do you really want to read that your surgeon went to a dinner party the night before your operation? You don't need the extra worry of "Did he drink alcohol or not last night?" as you prepare for your gallbladder operation on Monday morning. You have enough on your mind.

Furthermore, a social media site may expose your name to other patients and vice versa, which breaks the rule of patient confidentiality. Although the sites have features to hide a particular group of friends, mistakes can happen, and your identity could slip through. I also read an article where patients' opinions of their doctors were devalued when they discovered posts about their doctors' choice of cars and vacations. Remember, you're choosing your doctor on his ability to care for your health, not on how he chooses to spend his money and leisure time.

Communicating with Your Doctor in the Hospital

ICU: A Place Where Things Change Rapidly

The intensive care unit (or ICU) is a busy place. Patients are placed there for a number of reasons, including the following:

- When there is a need for minute-to-minute, hour-to-hour monitoring, such as right after an operation
- When the condition at hand could rapidly change, necessitating immediate attention by a nurse or doctor, such as with intestinal bleeding
- When there is a need for a vital procedure such as a central intravenous line placement into the chest or intubation (placing a tube into the windpipe to allow breathing)
- When the diagnosis at hand is life-threatening, such as a heart attack

Doctors round on their patients in the hospital once or twice a day and stay in touch all day with the nursing staff for critical updates.

Illnesses dealt with in the ICU are inherently unpredictable. Hence if your father is in the ICU with heart failure, and you ask the nurse how he's doing, she may say, "He's progressing nicely." You could ask her the same question in the afternoon, and her reply might be, "He's not doing so well."

When I was a resident, one attending doctor taught us never to give optimistic news to patients and their families while the patient is in the ICU. As residents, we were thrilled to report to our attending when our patients were improving—when, for example, they were liberated from the respirator or when a lab value improved from abnormal to normal. These results seemed like big victories to us, but the attending soberly reminded us of the big picture: "Remember, as long as the patient is in the ICU, their condition is serious and critical." He didn't want us giving the patients and their families hope until they were far removed from the ICU and getting ready to be discharged home.

So remember, if a loved one is in the ICU, he isn't out of the clear until he's out of the ICU with its constant monitoring by the nursing staff and the wired components attached to his body. A patient's condition is "critical" by virtue of being in the ICU. Nevertheless, keep notes on what the plan of the day is, if any procedures are scheduled, and the names of the different consultants who come to visit. Speaking of consultants, it is not unusual for one ICU patient to have multiple doctors come to visit. There may be an intensivist (who is also a lung specialist), a heart specialist, and an infectious disease specialist, not to mention others. If they have differing views on the course of action, that's OK. That's why they were called in. The head doctor in charge needs to gather various opinions in order to formulate a single treatment plan.

And even that plan may change. Everything in the ICU is tentative.

How to Communicate with Your Doctors on the Hospital Ward

All the same rules from the ICU in the previous section apply here, except that the pace is slower on the ward.

The Secret World
of Doctors

The Truth about Doctors

The truth is all doctors are busy. They are doing a lot more than meets the eye. They do much more than just meet face-to-face with patients in a clinic.

I divide my time into three jobs: (1) attending to patients in the clinic, about twenty to twenty-five per day; (2) returning phone calls and pharmacy requests, about twenty a day; and (3) attending to my patients in the hospital. I may have only about one to three patients in the hospital and a few more in the nursing homes, but when I take calls from the nurses or specialists, I have to immediately drop everything and take the call.

Plus there's more. My colleague has a framed sign for patients to comprehend exactly what they're paying for when they make him their doctor. It reads . . .

> Your fee is based on the time I spend with your during your visit, the complexity of your medical condition, and any treatment I provide. But proper attention to your care also requires that I or members of my staff spend additional time beyond that which we spend with you in the office. Such time may be used to:
>
> • Create or maintain your permanent medical record.
> • Review, interpret, and document all lab test results and communicate those results to you.
> • Review current x-ray or scan reports, compare them with reports of previous scans, and, when the studies are abnormal, consult with the radiologist.
> • Consult via telephone about your case with referring or consulting physicians and other health care providers.
> • Prepare referral letters to additional specialists, as needed.

- Prepare patient educational materials.
- Conduct medical research relevant to your case.
- Communicate with pharmacies about your prescriptions.
- Complete insurance applications and claim forms. Conduct utilization review negotiations with hospitals and insurance companies.
- Review and manage hospital records.
- Draft letters of necessity to obtain medical services, instruments, or prescriptions that you need.
- Arrange for hospital admissions and follow-up consultations with nurses, attending physicians, and house staff.
- Draft reports and forms, including home health care orders and facility orders.

All these activities add to our cost of doing business.
Yes, we're busy.

Myths about Doctors

1. *Doctors play God.* Doctors don't play God anymore, except in life-and-death situations where you can't wait for decorum and decisions must be made in a second, as in a heart attack, a stroke, an emergency surgery, or a childbirth. In those cases, I would want a doctor to take decisive action with lightning speed. However, the paternalistic, omniscient image of the physician has been eroding over the last three decades by a number of factors: the powerful rise of insurers, the rapid dissemination of medical knowledge, the overreliance on technology for diagnosis, the rising complexity of diseases requiring a team approach to health care, and a general distrust of the health care industry when medical errors and recalled medications hit the news. Where I work, doctors who "play God"—meaning those who are arrogant, self-righteous, inflexible, and unwilling to see another point of view—aren't very popular with other doctors or patients and don't last very long.

   Some persons, however, want a godlike physician: Someone to rescue them from ills, big and small. They want someone to make their difficult decisions for them (e.g., to have surgery or not to have surgery). Or someone to organize their medical information for them ("I don't remember my meds. They're all in your chart."). Treating your doctor like god won't be helpful to you. Assume a shared decision process.

2. *They're all rich.* While many cardiologists and orthopedists currently command mid-six-figure incomes for performing angioplasties and hip replacements, for example, there are some doctors struggling to make ends meet. Some young docs leave medical school with student loans as high as $100,000. And some docs are out of a job.

3. *They all know about optimal health and wellness.* The key words here are optimal health. If your physical condition runs on a spectrum, there would be illness on one end, optimal health and wellness on the other, and normal and just getting by in the middle.

In medical school, we learn about what defines a normal healthy body (in the middle of the aforementioned spectrum) in the first two years of medicine, and the rest of our schooling and training is in identifying and treating disease. Most doctors get a paucity of hours on what constitutes proper nutrition, normal sleep, exercise, and vitamins and supplements. Doctors are experts on illness. There are some doctors with extra training in wellness under the rubric of integrative health, holistic health, or alternative health. Fitness trainers, nutritionists, body workers, and naturopathic practitioners, for example, are sometimes more knowledgeable on optimizing health—in other words, wellness.

My point is to see a physician for *illness*. See a physician or a practitioner trained in wellness or preventive health for optimal health.

4. *If I heard it on the news, then the doctor surely must know about it already.* Not necessarily. The public consumes health news from television, radio, the Internet, and Dr. Oz. Doctors consume health news from conferences, pharmaceutical reps, continuing medical education, and journals. Sometimes news for the public makes headlines before it is published in respected scientific journals.

5. *My doctor would make a good friend.* Your doctor may be good at being compassionate, observant, and direct. Those are nice qualities for a true friend to have. Friends, however, tend to have interests and blind spots similar to you. They also tend to favor being nice to you over being blunt. Friends can be subjective. They may not be professionally objective. Don't confuse your nice doctor with your nice friends. I get lots of invitations to go to patients' parties and dinners. I usually don't go to avoid blurring the lines.

Forms

Do you have forms to fill out?

Forms are tedious. We despise them, but we fill them out anyway.

Some offices these days now charge to have forms filled out. Some types of forms include those for the following:

- Sport physicals
- Extended time off from work
- Work restrictions
- Short-term disability
- Life insurance
- School medication records
- College physicals
- DMV physicals
- In-home social services
- Discounts from local electric companies
- Family and Medical Leave Act (FMLA)
- Handicapped placards
- Psychological assessments
- Preoperative clearances
- Boy Scout camp

These forms are not standard across all agencies. For example, in my town, two local high schools have two completely different sports physical-clearance forms. One requires only my signature. The other requires filling out a questionnaire, documentation of height, weight, blood pressure, physical exam abnormalities, and a record of vaccinations.

I recommend filling out as much of the form as reasonably possible before bringing it to your physician. Some forms such as the FMLA have to be renewed annually. I highly appreciate it when a patient brings a copy of last year's form along with the current year's form. I usually transfer the same old information with just a few minor changes.

If forms are tedious, formal letters on a letterhead by your doctor are egregiously tedious. Make it easy for your doctor. (Note that I personally compose all of my own letters, not my secretary.) Provide your doctor with a one-page typewritten draft or template with the salient bullet points. Your doctor will make modifications from there.

Here are some examples of letters I've been asked to write:

- A description of a father's parenting abilities for a custody case
- An appeal to an insurance company for coverage of a very expensive drug
- A request to allow a tenant to keep a cat for the patient's mental well-being
- A detailed ten-year summary of a mysterious medical condition. The summary was needed for the insurance to cover a consultation with a renowned specialist in Beverly Hills.
- A neurological assessment for a fourth-grade student's Individual Educational Program (IEP) team at school

In each case the more information in print the patient provided, the faster I was able to finish the letter and charge the patient *less*.

DO:

Provide as much written information as possible along with the form you want filled out. Provide a draft or template.

DON'T:

Ask for a formal letter when a handwritten note on a prescription pad will suffice.

Death

Most people are uncomfortable talking about death—especially their own. Death is the number two issue that humans fear. (Public speaking is number one. And getting a colonoscopy is number three, I think.) Death is final, mysterious, and sometimes unpredictable. It is one thing we know with certainty that we will all confront. Yet it is one thing fraught with so much uncertainty: "What will I feel? Will there be pain? How will I die? When will I die? What happens afterwards?"

Our relationship with our mortality determines how we live our lives. My spouse, for example, is staunchly practical with the whole subject. His will is done. He has life insurance. He wants to be cremated because a plot takes up too much space. He doesn't ruminate about the afterlife because there are no facts about it. It's no wonder he has a quote on the pin board above his desk. It reads, "'Practically perfect people never allow sentiment to muddle their thinking.'—Mary Poppins." With that kind of attitude, it's no wonder he is full of life at the crack of dawn and accomplishes more in one week than most people do in one month. He is as buoyant about life as Mary Poppins is supercalifragilistic.

My father, on the other hand, had a conflicted relationship with death. He didn't want to die but talked about his death all the time. He wanted me to be a doctor but wanted no doctor's help at the end of his life. He left few plans for his funeral or estate. I think he was afraid of death and, at the end, afraid of living. He was indecisive.

This chapter is not meant to unravel the mystery of death but to underscore that everyone will one day pass away. I haven't met anyone immortal yet. Thus, the least that you can do is to prepare an advanced directive for health care. This legal document outlines to your doctor and your loved ones what kind of medical intervention, and to what degree, you would like to have in the event that you cannot communicate your wishes, especially if death is imminent. Such a document is a

71

gift to your caregivers. It designates who can speak on your behalf. It spares others the burden of making life-and-death decisions. It obviates second-guessing your medical requests. It can obviate divisive family disputes. It can ameliorate feelings of loss, regret, and guilt. It can save your family a protracted, agonizing, and costly death. (Forms according to your respective state can be found at http://www.caringinfo.org.)

The more specific your wishes, the less confusion there will be. Some patients in the ICU say that in the event of an emergency, "I want everything done." However, "everything" is vague terminology. Does "everything" include rib-fracturing cardio-pulmonary resuscitation even if there is no hope for recovery? Does it mean giving intravenous fluids or nutrition through a feeding tube if you are comatose? And for how long? A Physician Orders for Life-Sustaining Treatment (POLST) document defines what basic medical interventions you want done to save your life and your dignity. The form specifies which medical treatments you want and don't want when you are in a critical state. I recommend filling out a form together with your doctor. An example of a POLST form from California can be found at https://www.cdph.ca .gov/programs/LnC/Documents/MDS30-ApprovedPOLSTForm.pdf.

Doctor Euphemisms, or "I Don't Know, I'm Not God"

The one phrase doctors all doctors are embarrassed to say is "I don't know."

Most doctors won't deliberately withhold vital information from you. There may be a few exceptions, however. If you tell the doctor that you don't want to hear about a diagnosis, they might honor that request. Or in the case of an emergency or tragic outcome, sometimes the medical staff at a hospital will call you at home and say, "Please come to the hospital immediately. It's urgent." They won't tell you what's wrong until you get there. Why? Because disclosing the details may derail your focus while driving and cause you to be in a car accident.

The most difficult thing for a doctor to say is "I don't know." We've spent so much time, money, and effort expanding the limits of what we know and pushing the limits of scientific knowledge that we feel it's our responsibility to know. Saying "I don't know" feels inadequate and smacks of failure, although the reality is that medical science has yet to uncover many more mysteries.

Instead of withholding information, some doctors may use euphemisms that soften the blow. I've used some of them and I've seen them used in peer-reviewed journals, too.

What the doctor says	Translation
I'm concerned.	I'm worried.
I recommend.	I want you to do this.
obese	fat
Thank you for your patience.	I'm sorry to keep you waiting.
You will, most likely . . .	You will, but nobody knows when.

What the doctor says	Translation
That's a good question!	I don't know!
That's a great question!	I really don't know!
I apologize.	I'm sorry.
It's unfortunate.	It's sad.
I'm running behind.	You're taking too long.
Research shows . . .	See, I'm not the only one who thinks this.
I can help you stop smoking.	Stop smoking.
intimate relations	sex
having multiple partners	promiscuous
expire	die
nutrition or sustenance	diet
Please get active.	Please get your butt off the couch.
flatulence from above	burp
flatulence from below	fart
we (as in the royal "we")	you
we	we
inebriated	drunk
socioeconomic status	rich, middle class, or poor
MSM	men who have sex with men, regardless of how they self-identify
More research is needed.	Even the researchers don't know.
I'll read up on that and let you know.	I don't know.
poor judgment	mistake
That's outside of my specialty. Ask your primary doctor.	I don't know.
That's outside of my specialty. Ask your primary doctor.	That's outside of my specialty. Ask your primary doctor for legal reasons.
I don't know. Ask your specialist.	I don't know.
God knows.	I don't know.
There's always a risk.	Accidents happen.
complication	something that could go wrong

Bedside Manner Is in the Eye of the Beholder

Every year I approach my tax accountant with a stack of meticulously organized papers. I have my expenses and deductions clearly organized on a chart just like a diabetic listing his blood sugar readings. As if it's a doctoral thesis, I have spent hours making this chart that I hand over to my accountant. Instead of getting a pat on my head, he grabs it like a bunch of paper towels, scowls at it for ten seconds then puts it in a pile of receipts. I sulk inside.

Now I know how some patients feel when they say, "I brought the doctor what he wanted then he didn't even look at it. How rude!" Objectively speaking, my accountant did indeed look at it. He wasn't rude. He saw what he needed to see, made an analysis, and then moved on. If I had his years of experience, I probably would have done the same thing. Let's turn the tables. If my accountant brought me a chart listing his blood sugar readings and blood pressure readings neatly organized over the last month, with my experience I probably would need about ten seconds to read and analyze it. I would still thank him for the time he took to compose this chart. But the point is this: The client and professional may see different things on the same sheet of paper. Don't be offended.

One of the most common complaints I hear when a patient is disgruntled with a doctor is, "He might be good at what he does, but he has no bedside manner." My mechanic has no bedside manner—or carside manner. He listens with a drab face and then takes my car keys. He returns an hour later, my car fixed. He ekes out a quick explanation of the problem then hands me the bill. He still doesn't smile after I pay him—no social skills at all.

But I don't care. I'm not there for his social skills. I'm there for his auto mechanic skills, and his skills are great every time.

But since health care deals with your body and feelings, most people want a doctor who takes her time to listen, to explain, and to treat as gently as possible. Other than that, bedside manner is quite a subjective matter. For example, one study showed that patients who were interrupted by the physician before two minutes into their visit perceived their doctor as rude. They also perceived that their time spent with the physician was too short. Patients who were interrupted after two minutes, however, had perceived their doctor as a good listener and felt that their time spent with the doctor was adequate.

What determines that a bedside manner is good is quite subjective. Only one doctor's office I visited asked on the new patient questionnaire "How would you like the doctor to explain things to you?"

- In technical terms
- In layman's terms
- As brief as possible
- Not at all

The doctor here was a veterinarian.

With my new patients, I sometimes ask what they are looking for in a physician. Here are some of the answers I have received:

Someone who explains things clearly.
Someone who speaks English really good [*sic*].
Somebody nice.
Someone who believes the doctor is right.
Someone who believes the patient is right.
Someone who doesn't give shots!
Someone who returns my calls.
Someone who is thorough and orders tests.
Someone who does not order a lot of tests.
Someone who will reassure me.
Someone who will tell it to me bluntly.
Someone who will tell it to me kindly.

If the physician doesn't ask what kind of bedside manner fits you, I suggest you kindly tell them what you're looking for early on.

Work-Up

"Work-up" is medical jargon for "investigation." It means the series of tests and/or procedures that a doctor is planning. Tests may include blood tests, urine tests, x-rays, ultrasounds, CT scans, MRIs. It may include getting a biopsy (a piece of tissue taken from your body to be examined under a microscope). It may also include more sophisticated procedures, such as an endoscopy or an angiogram—an x-ray during which dye is injected into the blood stream to illuminate and delineate an artery, an organ, or a tumor in the body.

Tests are performed for a variety of reasons, for example:

- To confirm a diagnosis (rule in a diagnosis)
  For example, "Our *work-up* shows that the final diagnosis is indeed cancer."

- To exclude a possible diagnosis (rule out a diagnosis)
  For example, "The *work-up* does not show any evidence for an infection in the bloodstream."

- To provide more information in order to make a diagnosis
  For example, "It's unclear what your diagnosis is. We need a *work-up*."

When to Switch Doctors

WHEN TO SWITCH DOCTORS AND WHEN NOT TO

Today I met two different patients in urgent care. Joey needed to switch to a new primary doctor but didn't want to. Betty wanted to switch but shouldn't.

Joey was a thirty-year-old man who had been suffering from severe disabling arthritis. For the last six months, he had bouts of pain and swelling in his knuckles, ankles, and knees. During these bouts he was unable to drive, go to work, or care for his children. He could not take nonsteroidal anti-inflammatory meds due to a previous ulcer. His primary care physician (PCP) gave him tramadol and dumped his care onto a pain management specialist. The specialist was indignant that there had not been any prior work-up: No x-rays or blood tests. No evaluation with a rheumatologist. No explanation that arthritis of this severity was rare in someone his age and that pinpointing a diagnosis was crucial. The PCP did not return the specialist's calls or fax over any additional information. The pain management specialist remarked, "Usually patients come to me after all other treatments have been exhausted." The pain specialist felt that the primary physician shirked being thorough and responsible. Out of compassion and frustration, Dr. Pain Management took over the case completely, ordering and scheduling tests, referring Joey to a rheumatologist, and taking valuable time to call the insurance for prior authorizations on tests—actions usually undertaken by the primary doctor.

For six months, Joey had been suffering a disabling arthritic pain without a diagnosis and had been reduced from a thriving young husband to a man trying to tolerate his pain from day to day. He wanted to find another primary doctor but felt a switch would offend his current primary physician. "Does she care about you?" I asked. He said, "No, not really." "Then why do you care about her feelings, when she doesn't care about you?" He had no reply as he saw the illogic of placing his doctor's reactions over his own well-being. "Your health comes first," I said.

Betty was a 34-year-old entrepreneur who had seen many specialists before finally being diagnosed with thoracic outlet syndrome, a rare condition that can cause pain and weakness of the arm. She said her internal medicine doctor patiently collaborated with a neurologist and orthopedist to pin down the elusive diagnosis, after she was misdiagnosed by other specialists. Her only complaint was that her doctor was a thirty-minute drive from her new residence and she was looking for someone else closer. "I am so grateful for my doctor," she gushed. "Then why would you want to replace him with someone else? Are you telling me that you value local convenience over your body's well-being, especially after sifting through so many different doctors?" She paused and then realized a thirty-minute drive was a small price to pay for a doctor she trusted.

My patient Carl doesn't mind travelling to get the care he wants. He drives four hours across a desert to see me four times a year for his med evaluations and annual physical exam. He schedules his appointments with a rheumatoid arthritis specialist and a urologist on the same days that he sees me. He goes to an urgent care clinic near his home for acute issues like a badly sprained ankle. He was hospitalized two years ago for a serious skin infection on his hand that was treated at my local hospital, where his specialists are based.

Carl has carefully evaluated and created his system of care for primary, secondary, and tertiary care. He prioritizes having physicians he trusts and communicates well with over convenience and proximity. (Primary care includes well physical exams, preventive care, minor surgeries, and the first line of attention for common ailments. Secondary care refers to more sophisticated care provided by a hospital or specialist. Tertiary care is that provided by academic or university hospitals. It's where the doctors in secondary care refer to when they need help. Dr. House on TV is tertiary care.)

Clear communication emanating from both the patient and physician can facilitate rapport, continuity of care, and accurate diagnoses. However, even with clear communication, sometimes the doctor and patient may not be a good match. Perhaps the two of you may not agree on a treatment plan. Or perhaps the doctor personality's style (paternalistic versus collaborative) may not suit you. Or perhaps you're happy with the care you're receiving but are disappointed with the staff or vice versa. Or the doctor doesn't have the expertise in the condition you have. Whatever the reason, if you are not satisfied with the care you are receiving, especially after multiple attempts to rectify the problem, then seek another physician and have your medical records transferred.

A Very Short Glossary

There are hundreds of medical abbreviations that are used in spoken and written medical communication. This is by no means a comprehensive list. It is an alphabetical list meant to help you understand a few terms when conversing with your physician, watching a medical drama on television, or impressing your friends.

ABG: arterial blood gas

BID: twice a day

CHF: congestive heart failure

DNR: do not resuscitate

EtOH: ethanol (alcohol)

FEV1: force expiratory volume

GERD: gastro-esophageal reflux disease

H&H: hematocrit and hemoglobin

I&O: intake and output

INR: international normalized ratio

JRA: juvenile rheumatoid arthritis

KUB: kidney, ureter, bladder

LDL: low density lipoprotein (the "bad" cholesterol)

MRA: magnetic resonance angiography

NKA: no known allergies

OTC: over-the-counter

PE: pulmonary embolism

QID: four times a day

RSV: respiratory syncytial virus

SSRI: selective serotonin reuptake inhibitor (e.g., Prozac)

TIA: transient ischemic attack

UA: urinalysis

V/Q: ventilation perfusion (nuclear scan)

yo: years old

Zn: Zinc

Adapted from Taber's Medical Dictionary.

Appendix

HELPFUL RESOURCES ON THE WEB

Centers for Disease Control and Prevention.
   http://www.cdc.gov

U.S. Food and Drug Administration.
   http://www.fda.gov

MedlinePlus. U.S. National Library of Medicine.
   http://www.nlm.nih.gov/medlineplus

National Cancer Institute.
   http://www.cancer.gov

Mayo Clinic.
   http://www.mayoclinic.org

Cleveland Clinic.
   http://my.clevelandclinic.org/default.aspx

Bibliography

Anderek, William. "Should Patients Accept Gifts from Their Patients? Yes." *Western Journal of Medicine* 175 (2001): 76. Print.

Avitzur, Orly, MD. "How to Make Your Doctor Listen." *ConsumerReports.org.* Consumer Reports, May 2011. Web. 28 June 2013. http://www.consumerreports.org/cro/2012/04/how-to-make-your-doctor-listen/index.htm.

D., Dr. "Delayed Gratitude." *Ask an MD*, 26 Apr. 2010. Web. 29 June 2013. http://askanmd.blogspot.com/search?q=delayed+gratitude.

Gaufberg, Elizabeth, MD. "Should Physicians Accept Gifts from Patients?" *American Family Physician* 76.3 (2007): 437–38. Print.

Weijer, Charles. "Should Patients Accept Gifts from Their Patients? No." *Western Journal of Medicine* 175 (2001): 77. Print.

"What Doctors Wish Their Patients Knew." *ConsumerReports.org.* Consumer Reports, Feb. 2011. Web. 29 June 2013. http://www.consumerreports.org/cro/2012/04/what-doctors-wish-their-patients-knew/index.htm.

About the Author

Glenn Miya, MD, is a double-board certified physician in pediatrics and internal medicine, as well as a television and radio host, producer, writer, and speaker on current topics in the world of medicine and wellness.

His radio talk show *Smart Health* on the Star World Wide Radio Network brings together medical experts, authors, and patients to examine what works and what doesn't in staying healthy.

He was a television host for KVCR, a PBS affiliate in Southern California where he is in private practice. Dr. Miya is a member of the American Academy of Pediatrics, the American College of Physicians, Mayo Clinic Social Media Network, and Toastmaster's International.

www.ingramcontent.com/pod-product-compliance
Lightning Source LLC
Chambersburg PA
CBHW071243020426
42333CB00015B/1600